Starting your natural hair journey from scratch: Transitioning from relaxed to natural hair

Dr. VICTORIA EYOG TANG NLEND

DEDICATION

I dedicate this book to my mom, Eyog Njoki Christine for taking care of my natural hair throughout the years with lots of love, for letting me start the journey of relaxing my hair and for supporting me when I chose to revert to natural hair. Mom, the way you care for your hair inspired me to care for mine. I love you and I dedicate this book to you.

CONTENTS

ACKNOWLEDGMENTS

My acknowledgements go to the following people, who contributed in one way or another for this book to be written:

- My lovely husband, Dr. Louis Serge Tang Nlend who has always loved my natural hair and always encouraged me to remain nappy
- My Mom, Christine Eyog Njoki who always cared for my hair by putting it in protective hairstyles so as to limit damage
- My elder sister Dr. Rose Eyog for opening my eyes to the fact that it was possible for an African woman to grow long natural hair
- My aunt Dr. Leyla Olatoundji Siyam who made me realize that there were many black-skinned women on Youtube with type 4c hair just like me who had tips on how to manage their hair and make it grow
-Wolfgang Lisborg, the waves king, who taught me how to finesse my hair, who helped me to transition from relaxed to natural hair, who taught me that my hair doesn't have to break a comb and that combing natural hair doesn't have to be painful

You've all inspired me to write this book. May God bless you abundantly.

1 MY HAIR STORY

Hey there, my name is Victoria Eyog Tang Nlend. I am an African woman, born in Cameroon. I'm 28 years old writing this book and I have natural type 4c hair. Throughout my childhood, my hair was 100% natural. I would observe women from afar who had relaxed hair and I would envy them. This was because most of what I watched on TV showed me white or Asian women with long straight hair. As such, I deeply desired to have straight long hair. Mom's hair was relaxed. She knew the dangers and the side effects better than me. For this reason, she didn't want me to make the same mistake.

As soon as I reached high school, I convinced Mom to buy me a hair straightening iron. I was so fond of it. I used to straighten my hair with it every two weeks and to have the illusion that I was a Caucasian woman. After some months, it damaged my hair and my mom kindly helped me to choose between straight damaged hair and healthy kinky hair. That's how I ended up putting a break on straightening my hair.

As I entered first year university, I noticed that almost all the other girls my age relaxed their hair and used wigs or hair extensions. I was left aside as the minority which didn't relax her hair. I looked like an outcast. Most people called the other girls beautiful while I was considered like a "baby". I had long hair but I couldn't enjoy leaving it out like white women or like the other girls with relaxed hair. My hair was always in braids, cornrows or African threading. At that time, I had an inferiority complex towards my hair. I thought natural 4c hair wasn't beautiful. I believed it was too hard to manipulate especially considering the fact that despite doing a hair mask every month, my hair was generally dry, it was painful to comb and at times my hair would even break my comb teeth.

Finally, in year 2 of university, my mom accepted to relax my hair. I was so happy. My hair was silky and shiny.

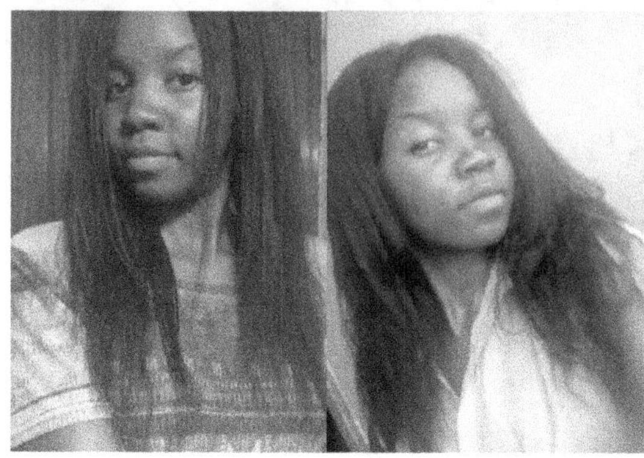

Relaxed hair plus Brazilian keratin treatment, April 2015

I thought I would be able to do like all the white girls in movies and just leave my hair out every day. I was very wrong. Relaxed hair required even more care and even more protection. It felt so fragile, so brittle. I had to do hair masks more often than usual, and of course the part I didn't expect, as new natural hair grew it became more and more difficult to comb all the hair and there was breakage at the junctions.

A friend of mine, Dr. Caroline gave me awesome tips on hair masks and how to stretch relaxers, and I even ended up doing Brazilian keratin treatment immediately after each relaxer session so as to straighten my hair. Nevertheless, my curly 4c texture would still grow back at the roots (normally) and the already relaxed hair wouldn't remain so straight as months went by (since I used medium strength relaxers).

I was always in the middle of two textures, so I still had to keep my hair in braids, twists or cornrows most of the time. It was very annoying. Most people would tell me "You have long hair, why don't you just let it out in the wind" but no matter how I explained to them that my hair would get puffy and frizzy and that the two textures would be visible, they wouldn't understand.

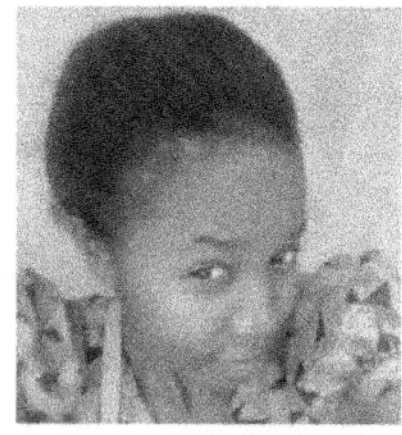

Thinning edges caused by chemical relaxers, Dec 2015

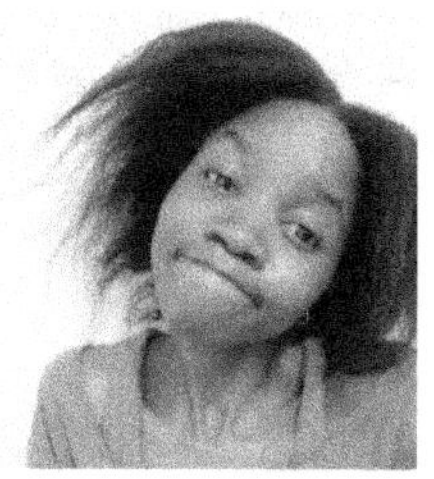

Breakage caused by chemical relaxers, March 2020

Then came the natural hair movement, and I was so admirative of the girls who reverted to natural. One of my aunts, aunt Leyla was 100% natural and even encouraged me to look for the best products for my hair. Yet I was skeptical of the natural hair movement because I knew my hair, I was so sure that it would break combs once more and be so painful to comb. All that was till the day I watched a video of nekicakes on YouTube who shared about Wolfgang Lisborg the Instagram waves king.

This man had long natural hair and he had techniques to "finesse" hair. Brother Lisborg became my hair coach for a few months. He taught me how to comb my hair without feeling any pain, without causing hair breakage, and without breaking any comb. He gave me techniques to moisturize my 4c hair. I was so grateful to God for enabling me to meet him. Thanks to his coaching I developed the courage to revert to natural hair. I didn't big chop immediately, I transitioned little by little. Then when I was ready to cut off the relaxed hair, I watched a YouTube video on the Rezo cut and that's how I cut off my relaxed hair. I reverted back to natural in 2021 and it has been an amazing journey since then.

Never again has it been painful to comb my hair. Never again have I broken a comb in combing my hair. People who see my natural hair love it and most importantly I love it too. By God's grace I've learned to love my hair and manage it in such a beautiful and respectful way for it.

I'm writing this book for women out there who may think that their natural hair isn't beautiful enough, who don't know how to manage it, who want to transition from relaxed to natural hair or who are already natural but aren't enjoying it yet. In this book I'll teach you how to gain mastery over your hair texture and how to love and enjoy your hair. Stay tuned and have fun.

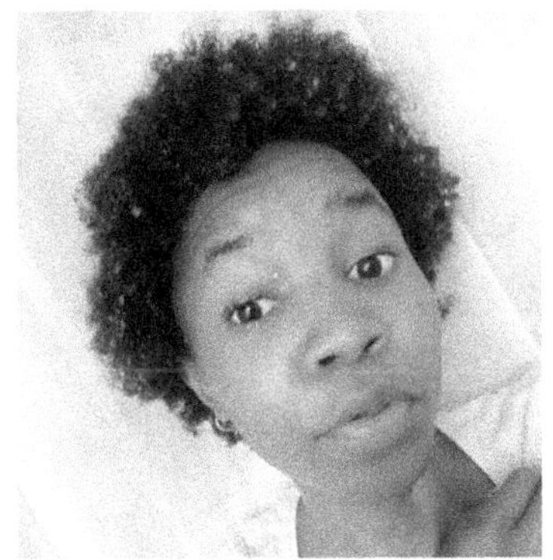

Big chop, June 2020

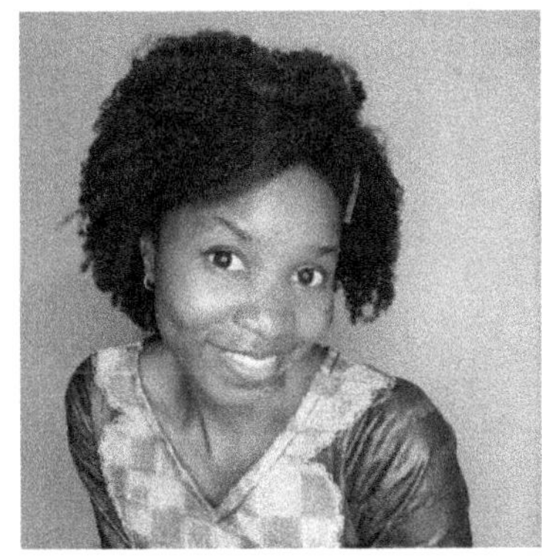

Healthy natural hair, June 2021

2 WHY WOMEN CHOOSE TO RELAX THEIR HAIR

Most women choose to relax their hair for some of the following reasons:

- **To keep it manageable:** As in my story, I thought my hair was normally hard and dry. Combing it was painful and difficult so I relaxed my hair to make it easy to comb, easy to manage
- To style their hair faster
- **To look like other women, to fit in, to be socially acceptable:** When you live in a community where everyone relaxes their hair, you'll easily want to relax your hair too so as to fit in. On the other hand, I noticed that there are tribes in our country Cameroon (mostly the Northern tribes) where women don't relax their hair at all nor wear extensions. Natural hair is considered beautiful so the women don't really have any peer pressure to relax.
- To feel more beautiful
- **They can't find hair salons specialized in natural hair**: the inability to find a hair Salon or at least a hair stylist specialized in natural hair leaves all the work to women to care for their natural hair. With time, many get tired of doing all those efforts and choose to relax their hair
- **Natural hair products are expensive:** Let's be true, natural hair products aren't as many on the market as other hair products. They're made with more care and more natural ingredients specifically for us the natural girlies. As such, they're more rare and more expensive. Many women can't afford to buy all those products as such they end up relaxing their hair, hoping to save money.

3 DANGERS AND SIDE EFFECTS OF RELAXERS

I can't deny the fact that relaxing hair has some advantages. It makes your hair more manageable, shiny, and in some cases, it even makes people to respect you more. Nevertheless, there are many associated dangers. Before sharing the general side effects that can be found on every website, I'll start by sharing the side effects that I experienced myself when I used to relax my hair and also what I observed when looking at other ladies around me who relaxed their hair.

- **Hair became more fragile, more breakage occured:** Even though my hair looked shinier and more lustrous as soon as I relaxed it, it started getting more fragile. I would comb and there would easily be breakage

- **Thinning edges and bald edges:** In applying relaxers, a little amount is always applied to the edges last so that it won't destroy the hair and the edges are first coated with Vaseline so as to limit damage. Nevertheless, relaxers damage hair no matter how you do it. So, with time, edges started thinning out and breaking and eventually I developed bald spots.

- **Hair looks shorter the more you relax:** this one happens most commonly in Africa I believe because here women in hair saloons don't respect instructions on relaxer boxes. Normally when you relax hair consecutively, you should relax only the new growths not all the hair but here in Africa, most women in hair saloons will re-relax all your hair every time which causes more and more breakage. So, the first time a lady relaxes her hair it looks so long but by the time she's at her 4th or 5th relaxer session her hair is either same length as when she started or three or four times shorter because of continuous damage and breakage. What I used to do to maintain long relaxed hair was I would relax only the new growth as my mom taught me. Other ladies would be amazed at the length but when I told them to stop relaxing all their hair all the time they wouldn't listen.

Now other side effects which you'll see
- Some relaxers have been associated with different forms of cancer amongst which uterine cancer and breast cancer [1–5]
- Inhaling the fumes from relaxers can be dangerous for health. I remember the story of a woman in Cameroon who died in her bathroom

while relaxing her hair because she mixed the chemicals and the fumes released were poisonous for her. That's why my mom always told me to relax outdoors and not in my room

- Hair loss and delayed hair growth: Hair relaxers can cause scalp inflammation, damage to the shaft, and hair loss[6]. I didn't personally experience this one but I have a friend who did and I have many patients who did. At times the relaxer is left for too long or is just too strong for your hair scalp so it ends up burning it such that hair has a hard time growing back there. I have a friend to whom it happened and for more than five years she was unable to regrow hair consistently on a specific spot on her head. She's been wearing wigs ever since

Another side effect which is not related to physical health but to mental health is this: many women as soon as they start getting relaxers, it becomes like an addiction. They can't revert back to natural because they believe deep down that their natural hair is ugly. Despite balding, breakage, burnt scalp and delayed hair growth, they keep relaxing their hair because they're convinced that without that they're not beautiful, which is quite sad because over the years they accumulate more and more damage as well as a poor self-image.

4 HOW TO TRANSITION FROM RELAXED HAIR TO NATURAL HAIR

Transitioning from relaxed hair to natural hair has become a trending topic a few years ago when many women chose to ditch down their relaxers and go back to natural. Many women want to start this journey but they're overloaded with so much information from almost everywhere such that they don't know where to start or how to do it. Nevertheless, you've come to the right place, I'll explain the basics to you, every essential thing you need to do.

There are two ways by which you can transition from relaxed to natural hair, with or without a big chop

1.   Transitioning with a big chop

Basically, the big chop is a process whereby you cut off all your relaxed hair at once so as to start over. This is generally for the most radical women who want to change all at once. All you have to do is cut off all your relaxed hair and start over.

2.   Transitioning without a big chop

Here you'll keep growing your hair but you will act like you're stretching relaxers. If you were to relax for example next month, you choose not to relax your hair. You keep washing it, combing it and styling it till the natural hair reaches the desired length. You could trim the relaxed ends every month or when you reach your final desired natural hair length you cut off the relaxed hair. This way, you never got to have very short natural hair. This is the method that I used.

However, I have to add something here. Managing two textures at the same time (natural and relaxed) isn't easy. You'll have to do regular hair masks as least once every two weeks and to be very careful while combing because the demarcation line between the two textures is an ideal spot for breakage.

I can tell you that in my transition process I experienced lots of breakage though people didn't really notice it but I knew what was going on with my hair. It wasn't easy but when I finally made up my mind to cut off the relaxed hair, I did a Rezo cut all by myself and I was very happy with the results. I had my short curly afro but it wasn't too short. I could still do buns as I enjoyed because I intentionally waited for my hair to reach that length before cutting it.

5 KNOWING YOUR HAIR TYPE AND HAIR POROSITY

Most natural hair experts will tell you that everything around natural hair care revolves around these two things: hair type and hair porosity.

1.   Hair type

There are several hair types as seen in the images below:

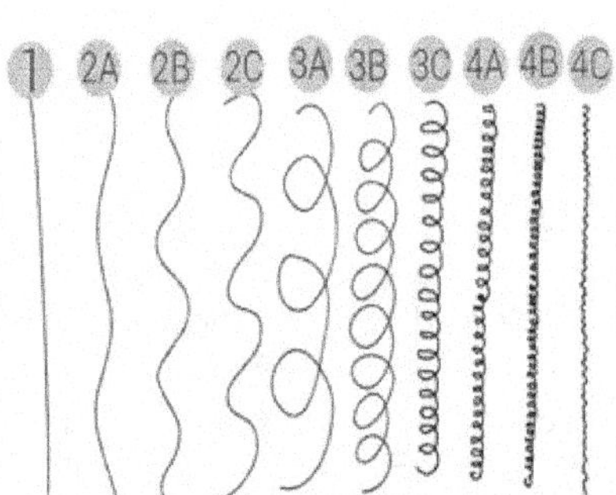

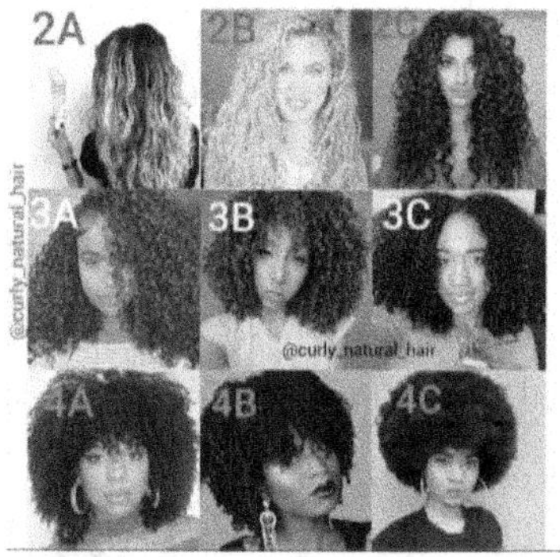

Hair types (@Hairyum, 2017)   Hair type chart (@curly_natural_hair)

My own hair type is 4C, the most kinky. Many African women are between type 3b and type 4. In fact it looks like most are even type 4. So basically, you determine your hair type based on the curl pattern that your natural hair makes.

2.   Hair porosity

Hair porosity has to do with how much water your hair can absorb and release back into the atmosphere and how fast

Low porosity hair (like my own) absorbs water difficulty, you have to wet it time and again for a long time for it to absorb water and it dries very fast. It's like the water just doesn't penetrate deep enough, same for products. That's why when your hair is low porosity you'll be advised to use heat when you condition your hair so that the product will penetrate through the hair and you're advised to use a sealant to seal in moisture and a humectant to absorb moisture from the atmosphere

High porosity hair on the contrary absorbs water so easily, it seem to be hydrophilic. It loves water and it also takes forever to dry. It generally looks more shiny and lustrous than low porosity hair and it has its own requirements which we'll discuss better later on in the chapter about maintaining hydration

Test for hair porosity [7] :

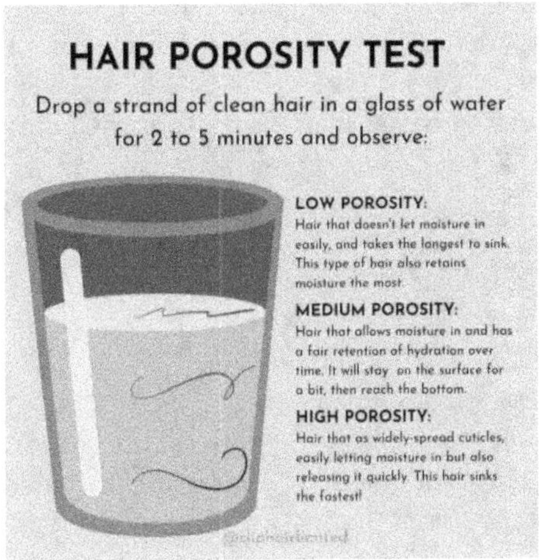

Test for hair porosity

Fill a glass of water and place a clean hair strand on it. If the hair sinks and goes to the bottom it is high porosity. If it remains in the middle, it is medium porosity hair and if it remains at the top it is low porosity hair.

6 HOW OFTEN YOU SHOULD WASH YOUR HAIR

I know that many hair gurus have different opinions about this. Some tell you to not wash your hair for a whole year claiming that shampoos damage hair. Others tell you to wash your hair every week but not with shampoo, they tell you to wash with conditioner. Some others say you can wash with shampoo but it has to be sulfate-free shampoo because shampoos which contain sulphates are too harsh for black hair.

In my own experience as a hair coach, I'll tell you to wash your hair at least once every two weeks. If you can wash once per week great but if you can't due to different hairstyles that you must maintain for at least two weeks try your best to wash your hair every two weeks

Why?
• Washing your hair enables you to get rid of dirt and excess oil build up.
• It makes your hair smell better
• It makes your scalp breathe
• If you have a good wash day routine it enables you to maximize hydration for your hair and the more your hair is hydrated the better

In reality there are two things that our hair type loves and needs a lot as taught to me by Wolfgang Lisborg. Water (lots of water) and vegetable oils. The more often you feed your hair on this the better

Now I told you about washing your hair once per week or once every two weeks but I didn't say it means you must wet your hair only once per week. Your hair thrives more if it's hydrated so ideally you should wet your hair every day. That's why we have DIY hair sprays. In fact, Wolfgang Lisborg wets (the waves king) wets his hair every single day. He will wet it in the morning in the shower with hot water and style it directly while it's wet and in the evening, he applies vegetable oils unto his hair. His hair grows like so fast with that. I wasn't able to maintain that rhythm because my scalp was just in pain when I manipulated my hair every day. So, I instead prefer doing twists and then spraying my hair with a hair tea to keep in hydrated every day.

7 CONDITIONING AND HAIR MASKS

Let's be real with each other. One of the reasons why many people think that natural hair is ugly is because they have the image of natural hair as dry and unkempt. Whereas when you condition/nourish your hair appropriately and it's well hydrated, when you go out of that home with that natural hair, everyone is in admiration and everyone wants tips from you.

You have to learn that it's not enough to just use shampoo. If you want beautiful natural hair, you must condition it and you must use hair masks.

This is what I generally do on a wash day: I start with a shampoo, then I use a natural DIY hair mask, something very messy eg. with avocado and eggs, then I leave the hair mask on for 2-4 hours, then I rinse it out and apply a store-bought conditioner and/or hair mask. I may or may not apply heat with my hair steamer but ideally, I apply heat, when possible, just so that the heat makes my hair to be saturated with the products. Then I rinse it all out and brush my hair with hot water and then I apply a hair butter and finally I style my hair (generally in twists). When I come out from there my hair looks so moist, so shiny and so happy

Note that I generally use only store-bought hair masks when I'm too busy for natural DIY hair masks.

Some DIY hair masks that I have personally tried and worked on for years:

1. **Avocado hair mask:** One ripe avocado, one egg and the oil of your choice (olive oil, coconut oil, fenugreek oil, carrot oil), one or two tea spoons of a hair growth powder of your choice (amla, fenugreek, henna, clove, spirulina). You may also add aloe vera gel, okra gel or flaxseed gel. Mix it all in a blender till it's smooth, apply it to your hair and let it rest for 2-4 hours. In order to shorten the time, if possible place your hair under a heat cap for some 20-45 minutes or use a steamer so as to ensure deep conditioning.

2. **Yoghurt hair mask:** One cup of yoghurt, one egg and the oil of your choice (olive oil, coconut oil, fenugreek oil, carrot oil), one or two tea spoons of a hair growth powder of your choice (amla, fenugreek, henna, clove, spirulina). You may add honey if you desire. You may also add aloe vera gel, okra gel or flaxseed gel. If your yoghurt is made

of soy, that's even better. I noticed that soy works wonders on my hair.

3. **Banana hair mask:** This mask defines my curls more than any other mask. Blend one banana, a teaspoon of honey, one egg and the oil of your choice. Apply as previously explained.

4. **Maize pap hair mask:** Take maize flour, add some water, mix it, till it's cooked pap. Let it cool down and then add one egg and the oil of your choice (olive oil, coconut oil, fenugreek oil, carrot oil), one or two tea spoons of a hair growth powder of your choice (amla, fenugreek, henna, clove, spirulina). Blend it and apply as explained above.

5. **Rice pap hair mask:** Take rice flour, add some water, mix it, till it's cooked pap. Let it cool down and then add one egg and the oil of your choice (olive oil, coconut oil, fenugreek oil, carrot oil), one or two tea spoons of a hair growth powder of your choice (amla, fenugreek, henna, clove, spirulina). Blend it and apply as explained above.

6. **Soy pap hair mask:** Take soy flour, add some water, mix it, till it's cooked pap. Let it cool down and then add one egg and the oil of your choice (olive oil, coconut oil, fenugreek oil, carrot oil), one or two tea spoons of a hair growth powder of your choice (amla, fenugreek, henna, clove, spirulina). Blend it and apply as explained above.

Some Hair masks and conditioners which you can purchase

Look out for ingredients like Shea butter, coconut oil, argan oil, cocoa butter etc. things with natural butters and vegetable oils. That's what you want in your hair. I will recommend a few brands of hair masks and conditioners that I know:

1. Shea Moisture
2. Soft Carrefour
3. Ultra Doux
4. Mielle
5. Tgin
6. Cantu

You can see a list of more than 20 of these products on my amazon storefront by clicking here on this link

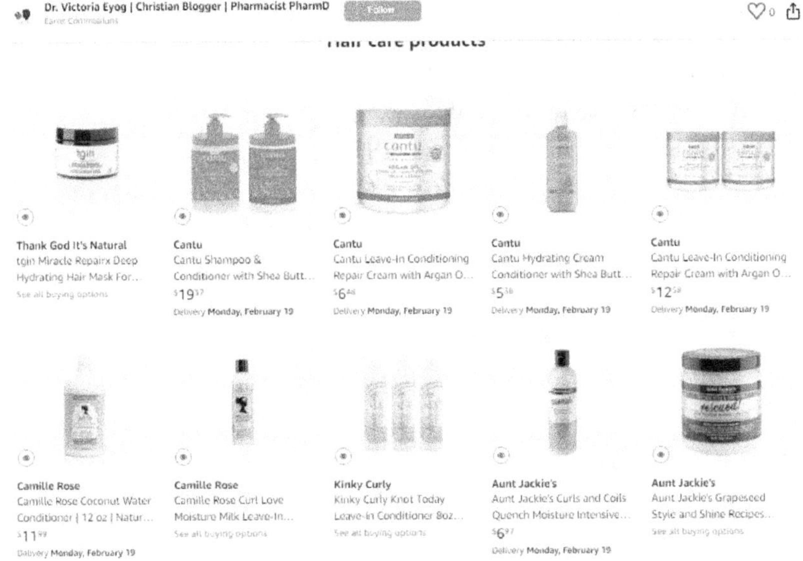

Deep conditioning:

This is a process whereby hair is strengthened and breakage is prevented by using a conditioner with ingredients which penetrate into the hair strand e.g. of such ingredients avocado oil, olive oil, hydrolyzed proteins.

Ensure to choose a conditioner labelled "deep conditioner", apply it to hair and leave it on for 20 minutes at least while being under a heat cap.

Deep conditioning your hair with heat will make it better such that your hair will remain moist and nourished for a longer time.

Once you're done let the hair cool down and rinse with cold water so as to seal the cuticles.

Protein treatments: There should be a moisture-protein balance for your hair. That's why you must moisturize your hair but you must also supply proteins to your hair.

Hair which is in proteins shortage lacks elasticity, the curls are lifeless and the hair breaks easily. You can find hair protein treatments in the store, many of those contain keratin or you can buy them or you can manufacturers them yourself by modifying the above recipes of hair masks by adding ingredients rich in proteins (for example eggs, soy bean pap). You can visit my amazon store front by clicking here on this link to find some protein treatments to purchase.

NB: When you have high porosity hair, you should do protein treatments at least once every two to three weeks while when you have low porosity hair you must not do frequent protein treatments. Once every 3-6 months may be enough. The biggest need of low porosity hair is regular deep conditioning under heat.

8 HAIR COMBS AND BRUSHES USED IN DETANGLING HAIR

A major reason why women relax their natural hair is because they find it way easier to manage when it's relaxed.

I remember how in childhood just the idea of having to comb or brush my hair would make me cry. It was always an extremely painful process. At times, my comb would even get broken in the process of combing my hair. As such, when I was thinking about reverting to natural hair the scary part for me was "how will I detangle my hair?". Fortunately for me, watching a Nekicakes Youtube video where she talked about the waves king Wolfgang Lisborg brought me to text him on Instagram and then brother Lisborg became my hair coach and taught me what I had to know about detangling tools. In this book, I'm gonna share with you his secrets which worked for me in this book.

1. Never detangle or comb your hair with cold water. Use hot water and it will be so much easier. Your hair must be not just damp but soaking wet in hot water.

2. Prior to detangling your hair, you should have applied a vegetable oil to it and let the oil seat overnight on the hair. The heat of the water will enable the nutrients from the oil to penetrate the hair shaft.

3. Don't start directly with a comb. Use a paddle brush (rectangular or circular). Hold it vertically and go through the hair. The brush will create spacing between the hair and detangle it. At this moment you can add conditioner if you wish to make it easier.

4. Don't start brushing from the roots. Divide your hair into sections, you can divide into two big sections (left and right) and then brush through the hair from the tips/ends then go up gradually little by little all that vertically so as to give a good wave/curl pattern.

5. Once you're done with the paddle brush you can comb the hair with a rake comb once more in sections and from the ends to the roots little by little. Keep adding more hot water because your hair has to be soaking wet.

6. The thing with combs is that you can go from a comb which has a lot of space in between its teeth to a comb which has less space progressively till you reach the fine-tooth comb. It will require patience, but it will get you rid of shed hair and it will give you a very defined curl pattern.

7. If you're not looking for a lot of definition you may skip the step of progressively going from one comb to another till you reach the fine-tooth

comb and you can go directly to styling your hair with a boar bristle waves brush.

8.   You can now use a special brush like a Denman brush to curl any part of your hair where you want to define those curls

Here attached are images of each brush.

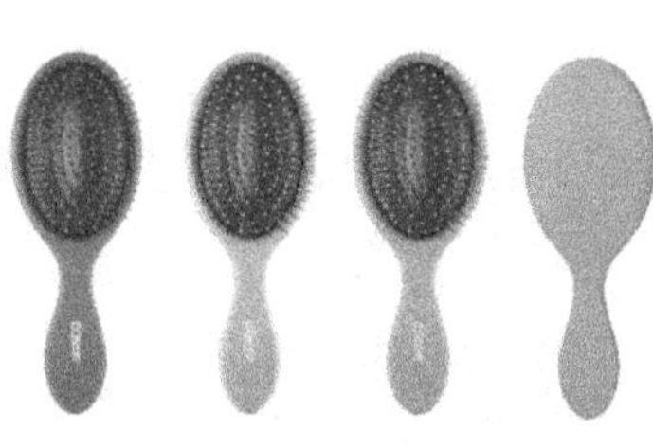

Oval-shaped paddle brush

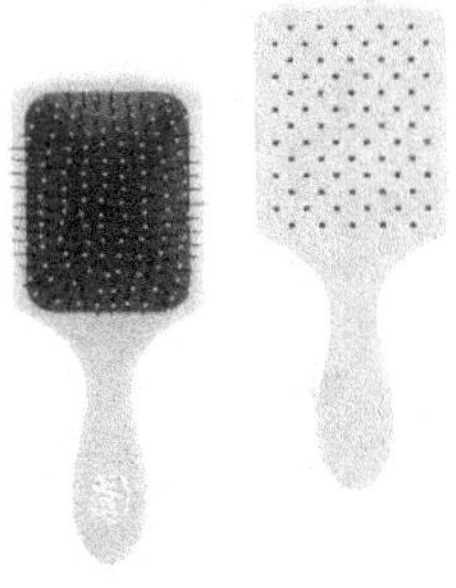

Rectangular-shaped paddle brush

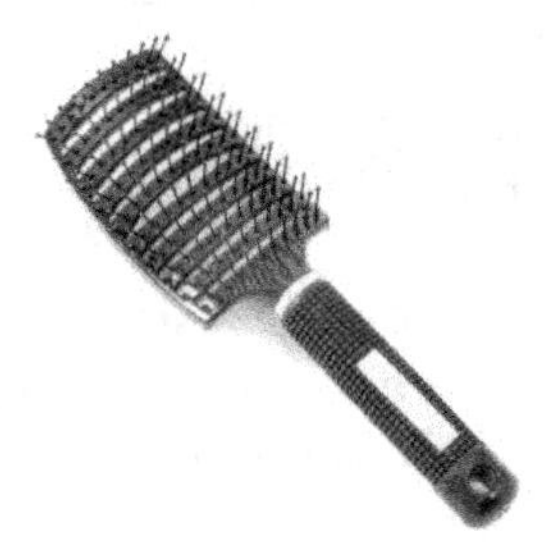

Detangling brush (my favourite)

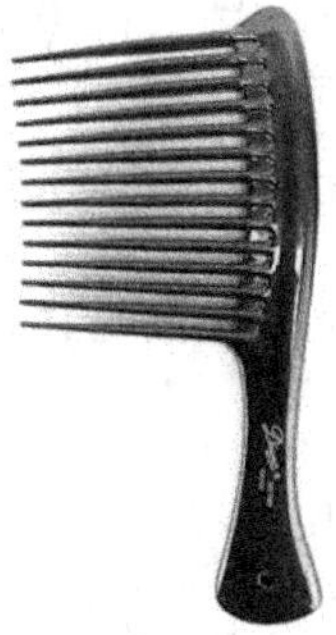

Rake comb

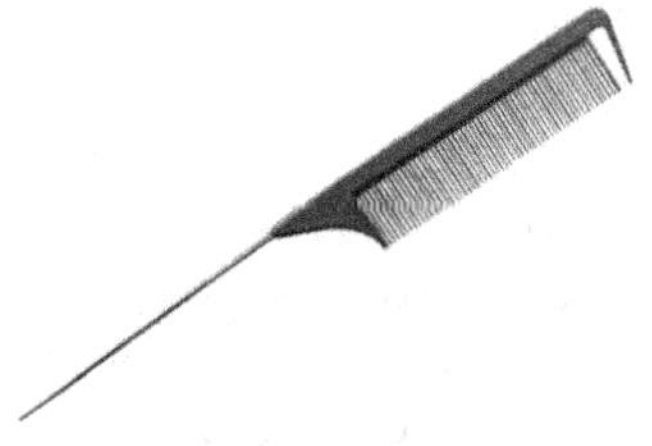

Fine tooth comb with pin tail

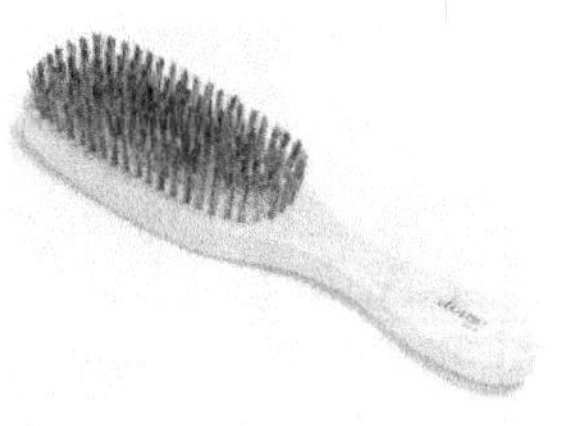

Boar bristle waves brush

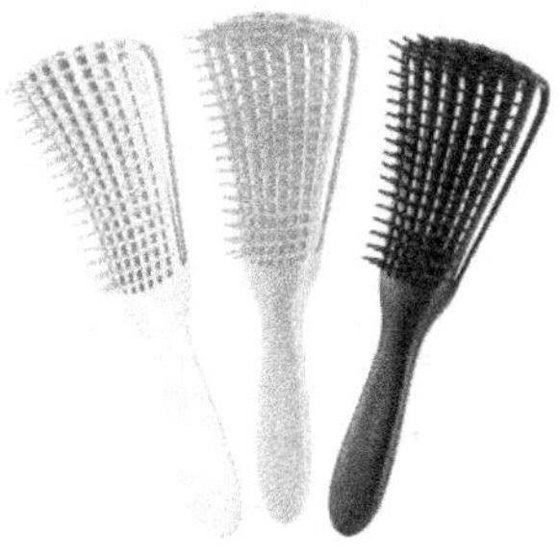

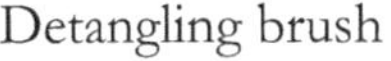

Detangling brush

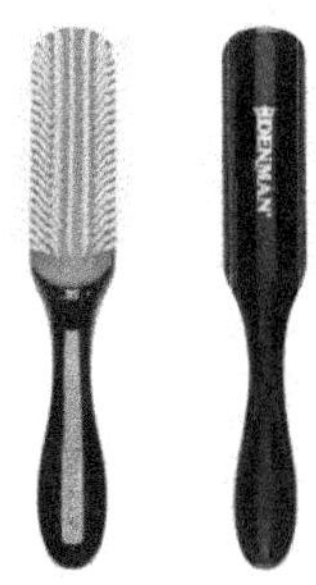

Denman brush to define curls

I know there are other many brushes which are advertised online. You may try them out and add them to your routine so long as you ensure that you're using hot water, a good conditioner and that your hair is soaking wet. You can get these brushes on my amazon store front by clicking here.

Dr. Victoria Eyog | Christian Blogger | Pharmacist PharmD
Earns Commissions

46 ITEMS • Updated today

Hair care products

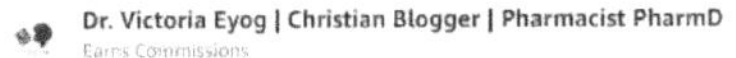

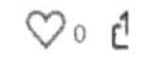

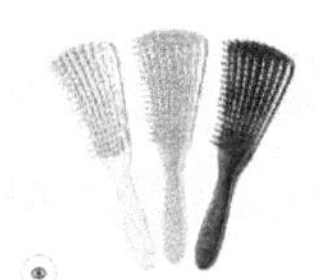

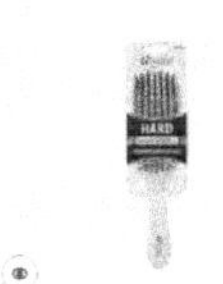

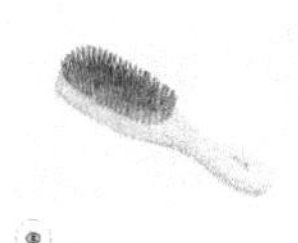

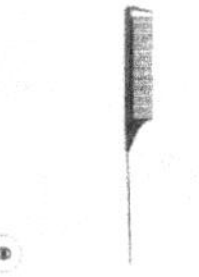

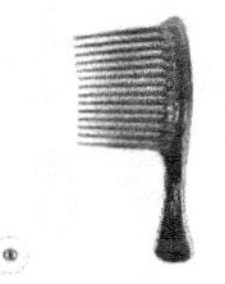

A.DASHER
3 Pack Detangler Brush for Natural Hair, Afro...
See all buying options

Annie
Annie Hard Wave Boar & Nylon Bristle Brush Light...
$7⁷²

Diane
Diane Reinforced Boar Bristle Wave Brush for Men and...
See all buying options

Diane
Fromm Carbon Fine Tooth Pin Tail Comb, 9.25 Inch
See all buying options

Diane
Diane RakeRage Comb BoneBlack, 1 Count, Hair.
See all buying options

9 DEFINING YOUR CURLS

The cutest part about having natural hair is the way it curls when you define your curls appropriately. What then can you do then to define your curls? You need the right tools and the right hair products.

Talking about the right tools, there are specific brushes like the Denman brush (shown in the previous chapter) which will enable you to define your curls. You can also use curling rods such as flexi rods and perm rods to curl your hair.
Talking about the right hair products, there are curling creams, curling custards, hair mousses which will help you achieve the type of curls which you want. You can find some of these products as well as curling rods on my amazon store front by clicking on the link here.

In order to define your curls, you'll have to use your curling products and your curling tools together.

NB: One thing which happened to me when I was trying to define my curls was that I would watch a video of a woman with 3c hair and try the curl-defining Denman brush on my hair and expect it to produce curls like the woman with 3c hair while it produced curls like the 4c hair woman that I am. If you want to watch tutorial videos on curling tools and curling products, watch the tutorials of people who have the same hair texture as you so that you won't be disappointed later on.
Now, if you're a 4c haired girl like me but at times you want curls which look very different from your curl pattern, there are a few things you can do.
1. Start with dry straight hair. Straighten your hair using either heat or not. As for me, I prefer not using heat, so I like stretching my hair using African threading method
2. Apply mousse to your hair and use curlers which will produce the desired curl pattern. (There are various shapes and sizes so that you can obtain the desired result)
3. Let the hair completely dry by air (it may take days in some cases) or under a hair dryer.
4. Take out the curlers and enjoy your curls for a few days. Note that as soon as the curls take in moisture from the atmosphere, they're going to change. In order to maintain your curls for a longer period of time, wear a satin hair cap or a durag to sleep, or use a satin pillow case.

10 PROTECTIVE HAIRSTYLES

If you want your natural hair to grow in a healthy manner, you must wear protective hairstyles.

When you're just from reverting to natural hair, it's tempting to want everyone to look at your hair, to try the fanciest hairstyles with natural hair, to try a new hairstyle every day or every two days and even to slay your edges daily with edge control.

The thing is the more you manipulate your hair and expose it to harsh environmental conditions, the more you can experience breakage. Reason why many naturals opt for protective hairstyles.

You can keep your hair in braids, twists, french braids, cornrows or African threading. You can style them and leave them for two weeks and renew the protective hairstyle every two weeks. While your hair is in a protective hairstyle you can spray it daily with hair growth teas before going out in the morning and you can apply hair growth oils on the roots and strands before going to bed. Afterwards, cover your hair with a satin scarf or hat or sleep on a satin pillowcase so as to maintain moisture in your hair and so as to not have the oils staining everything on your bed.

Now, for aesthetic reasons, many women will prefer doing braids and twists with hair extensions. I don't know if I'll still consider it as a protective hairstyle because the hair extensions are putting some form of pressure on your natural hair and depending on how long you keep the hairstyle or on how it was braided you may lose some hair because of that especially if you keep it on for months.

Nevertheless, I also noticed that there are some women in the natural hair community who will do cornrows or twists with their natural hair only and hide them under wigs. They'll do that for months. Some have even kept corn rows for 5-6 months, just ensuring that they didn't miss to wash their hair every week or every two weeks and that they didn't miss to spray hair growth tea every day and to apply hair growth oil everyday too. They've had tremendous growth because they didn't really manipulate their hair during that time but they also had a lot of accumulated shed hair.

I'm not so fond of wigs, for the moment I have only one wig and I prefer my natural hair and I don't braid a lot with extensions but it's up to you to experiment with those methods and see what works for you

What works for me is just twisting my hair and washing it every two-three weeks (max 4 weeks) so as to detangle it well and retwist while applying hair growth tea and/or hair growth oil daily. So that's my style.

The big conclusion here is you do you; you will experiment and find out what works best for you and from there you'll be thriving.

You could also decide to not go for protective hairstyles. Brother Wolfgang Lisborg for example isn't so much into protective hairstyles. He will do simple buns every day after hydrating and styling his previously oiled hair in the shower with hot water and conditioner every single day. The good thing is that all those oils plus the regular water supply will make your hair grow and the fact that you're brushing it and combing it daily will free you from tangles. I tried that for a while. Your hair will become even more shiny. Nevertheless, this is something to do if you have like 30 mins-1 hour every single day to give to yourself to take care of your hair. Not everyone can do that but it's a great method. If at all you do protective hairstyles like braids and twists, he advises to not keep them for too long as the hair will get dry and you may get breakage.

11 MAINTAINING HYDRATION: LOC, LCO AND THE MAXIMUM HYDRATION METHOD

What usually makes natural hair not to look beautiful in the sight of others is when it looks dry and unkempt. Maintaining hydration is key to have your hair always looking beautiful and lovely.

Here we'll discuss about three hydration techniques. The first two are based on your hair porosity.

1. LOC Hydration method

L.O.C stands for Liquid, Oil and Cream

So, after washing and conditioning your hair, after using hair masks, the very the last step is the L.O.C method if your hair is high porosity hair.

The Liquid: This could be water or liquid-based leave-in conditioner, it will hydrate the hair. The best liquid to use here is water because it is the number one source and only true form of moisture. It will penetrate the hair shaft and go deep into the hair's cuticle making your hair soft and supple.

Oil: Oil will help slow down the evaporation of water from the hair shaft. It should be a penetrative oil if your hair is high porosity eg. Olive oil, coconut oil, avocado oil.

Moisturising cream: The cream will add an extra layer of moisture and slow down the loss of moisture.

2. LCO hydration method

L.C.O stands for Liquid, Cream and Oil. It is adapted to low porosity hair.

For Low porosity hair, the moisturizing cream is used directly after the liquid and the last step is to use oil so as to seal hair to keep in moisture. Some natural hair girls even prefer to use a butter.

The best oils to use for this last step for low porosity hair are **sealant oils**. They do not penetrate the inside of the hair shaft; they sit on top of the hair and add shine or lustre. They seal in moisture (Sealant oils and butters are also ideal when you twist your hair).

Eg. Grapeseed oil, jojoba oil

NB: Shea butter is a sealant butter

3. **Maximum hydration method** [8]

Step 1: The Cherry Lola Treatment

As the first step in the Max Hydration Method, you'll want to create a mixture that's known as the Cherry Lola Treatment, which combines a number of ingredients to hydrate, reduce frizz, and make hair easier to detangle.

Recipe:

- 2 cups greek yogurt
- 2 tbsp baking soda
- 2 tbsp organic apple cider vinegar
- 2 tbsp raw coconut amino acids or regular amino acids
- 1/2 tbsp raw honey
- 1 tbsp unsulfured molasses
- 1/2 an overripe plantain or banana
- 3/4 tbsp avocado
- 1 egg (optional, but I used it no problem)

The mixture is to be applied to dry, detangled hair, saturating it from root to tip. Once each strand is evenly coated, put your hair up into a shower cap. You'll leave this on for between an hour and a half to two hours and then rinse thoroughly with warm water.

Step 2: Clarify

Clarify your hair with a baking soda rinse or use an apple cider vinegar rinse.

Baking Soda Mix: You'll mix one and a half tablespoons of baking soda into 1/3 a cup conditioner and let sit on the hair for ten to thirty minutes.

Apple Cider Vinegar Mix: You put in a spray bottle a 1:1 ratio of water and apple cider vinegar and spray on hair, leaving it for thirty minutes to an hour.

Step 3: Co-Wash

Since some shampoos can strip hair, co-washing is meant to cleanse while conditioning which is beneficial to natural hair types. You'll section the hair and apply your co-wash product from root to tip, apply a shower cap, and steam the hair for twenty minutes. You can checkout good steamers by clicking on the link here.

Step 4: Bentonite Clay Mask

The Bentonite clay mask makes the curls pop. Depending on your hair's needs, you can mix the clay with honey and an oil of your choice. I generally use Kaolin clay instead of Bentonite Clay because Kaolin clay is more easily available in my country, Cameroon than Bentonite clay. You can purchase clay by clicking on this link here.

Ingredients:

- – 1 cup bentonite clay
- – 1.5 cups of warm water or some apple cider vinegar
- – 1 tbsp of honey
- – 1 tbsp of olive oil

Clay masks can be messy in general, so applying it to the hair will likely result in a mess. To ensure you get the benefits, you'll want to separate the coils as you go and apply the mask in thin layers to prevent the hair from tangling or clumping together. You'll leave this on for at least 15 minutes.

Step 5: Apply Your Styling Products

Leave-in Conditioner: For this step, you'll want to do in the shower or under running water to ensure the hair gets all of the water it needs. Apply it in sections running it through from root to tip to ensure you get out any tangles.

Gel or Creme: Now, you'll apply your gel or creme in sections. To achieve elongated, defined curls, you may prefer to use a gel as cremes seem to just sit on top of hair for some people. Once you've applied your gel of choice, turn your head over and give it a big shake from side to side and up and down to separate your curls without touching them to prevent frizz. (Examples of natural gels you can use are Okra gel, Flaxseed gel, Aloe vera gel)

Step 6: Stretch your curls

If you're truly washing-and-going, you'll follow the same steps of shaking the hair out, using a diffuser to cut down your drying time. To diffuse with optimal results, 4c hair types should keep the blow dryer on the lowest setting (and don't touch your hair with your fingertips, which creates friction and, subsequently, frizz). To get more volume, flip your head over as you dry with the diffuser, shaking hair out at the roots rather than touching or running fingers through it.

If you're doing this before getting ready for bed and want to air dry, you can stretch your hair by using the Banding Method. You'll part the hair into four or more sections (depending on your hair's thickness and texture). Start by securing each section with an elastic band. Be careful not to tie too tightly as we want to keep our edges and coils in place. Elastic bands or silk scrunchies are ideal because they will secure the hair without snagging.

Finally, you'll take another band and weave it down the length of each ponytail to the ends of the hair. Now, it's time to secure your ponytails with a silk scarf or bonnet.

Note that the Cherry Lola Treatment is recommended to do every two weeks, while the rest of the steps within the Max Hydration Method should be done weekly to maintain hydration and moisturization.

NB: I read some YouTube comments which said you should use the deep conditioner after the clay and that your hair will feel better afterwards

12 HAIR OILS AND HAIR BUTTERS

The best oils for you will depend on your hair porosity

The best oils for Low porosity hair are:

-        Argan oil: forms a protective layer of moisture over the hair

-        Grapeseed oil: light texture, seals in moisture without weighing hair down

-        Jojoba oil: easily absorbed, texture similar to natural sebum

-        Baobab oil: contains linoleic acid which retains moisture

-        Sunflower seed oil: light and easily absorbed by the hair

-        Avocado oil: is heavier than the other oils but can penetrate the hair deeply so as to moisturize it

It's advised not to use coconut oil on low porosity hair because its molecules are too large and it won't let water molecules enter the hair shaft thus leaving the hair dry.

The best oils for high porosity hair are:

- Castor oil
- Coconut oil
- Olive oil

The best oils for normal porosity hair are:

- Black seed oil
- Grapeseed oil
- Neem oil
- Rosehip oil

Some hair butters:

- Cocoa butter
- Shea butter
- Mango butter

You can use these butters to seal in moisture into the hair especially when you style your hair in a protective style like braids

This is what I recommend that you do:

- Have a hair oil (it can be a combination of several hair oils) that you can use daily on your hair, it could be a hair growth oil

- Have a hair butter that you use to seal in moisture every time you style your hair in a protective hairstyle

The DIY Hair growth oil recipe I use:

- Rosemary leaves
- A carrier oil (eg olive oil, almond oil, sunflower seed oil)
- Hibiscus flowers
- Cloves
- Fenugreek seeds

Mix it all together. Let it sit for 1 month, strain it then start using it daily

If you're in a haste to use it you can put it in a water bath for 30 minutes, then let it sit overnight before straining it and using it

The DIY Hair Growth butter I use:

- Take 50% of your hair growth oil and mix it with 50% shea butter (or you can use a mixture of cocoa butter, mango butter and Shea butter). Start with all of it melted and cooled down in a freezer

- Blend or whip it for 30-45 mins

- Use it as desired for each protective hairstyle

13 DEVELOPING YOUR OWN HAIR REGIMEN

If you just read this book but you don't apply any of it, it will just be like a book you read but it won't produce results for you. It's time for you to select from all you've learned in this book and write down what you will do.

Open your journal and answer the following questions:

1.   What is my hair type?
2.   What is my hair porosity?
3.   How often do I want or need to wash my hair?
4.   What are the products that I will use on washday? (Shampoo, conditioner, deep conditioner, butter, oil, DIY hair masks etc.)
5.   In which order am I going to use these products?
6.   What are the tools that I will use on washday?
7.   In which order will I use those tools?
8.   What are my 1-3 go-to protective hairstyles?
9.   How often will I style my hair into protective hairstyles?
10. What care will I supply to my hair when it's under a protective hairstyle and how often?

If you answer these questions and you stick to it, it will help you to develop your own good hair regimen. You'll be able to observe what works with you and what doesn't work and to improve it with time and experience

Sample answer
1.   Type 4c
2.   Low porosity
3.   Once every two weeks
4.   Shampoo and conditioner containing Shea butter, deep conditioner, water, leave-in conditioner, Shea butter
5.   After shampoo, conditioner and deep conditioner under a plastic cap or heating cap I'll use Liquid, Cream, Oil or butter
6.   Paddle brush, rake comb
7.   Paddle brush, rake comb
8.   Twists and braids
9.   Every two weeks
10. Spraying with a hair tea in the morning and applying hair growth oil at night

14 HAIR GROWTH AND MAINTENANCE

In this section I'll tell you about the best tips which I know to grow and maintain long hair.

- Have a good hair regimen and stick to what works for you

- Never neglect deep conditioning (especially under heat)

- Avoid using gel on your hair all the time

- Don't slay your edges every day, it's dangerous and it may increase the chances of having balding edges

- Don't do tight buns all the time, it puts a lot of strain on your hairline

- Speak positively to your hair and to your body in general

- Don't wear only wigs and extensions, let your hair breathe most of the time

- Avoid relaxers, but if ever you relax your hair, never relax already relaxed hair. Touch up the new roots only

- Avoid dying your hair with chemicals, it causes damage. Instead opt for colored waxes, they're safer for your hair

- Detangle and comb hair progressively from the tips to the roots, not directly from the roots

- In order to avoid heat damage, use hair straighteners on your hair the least possible, once every six to twelve months maximum. Use hair protective sprays against heat damage when you use hair straighteners

- Avoid over manipulating your hair

- Avoid letting everyone touch your hair anyhow. *"Some people's hands aren't so good and when they touch your hair, they can cause growth stunt or damage"*

- Ensure that your hair receives enough protein and enough moisture

- Avoid those wigs that require using glue. It will damage your frontline very fast and make you bald with time

-        Take hair growth supplements for three months (Biotin, collagen, MSM). Some of my choice hair supplements are available on my amazon storefront, you can click on the link here

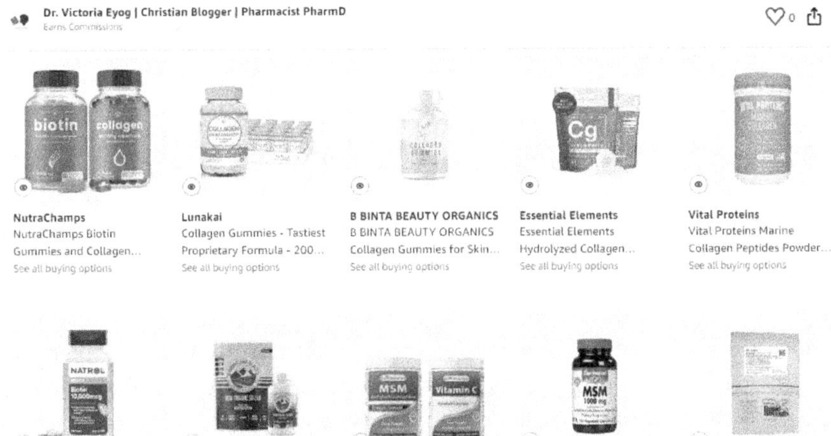

16 YOUR HAIR AS GOD'S GIFT TO YOU

'I will praise You, for I am fearfully and wonderfully made; Marvelous are Your works, And that my soul knows very well'

__ Psalms 139:14 NKJV

'But even the very hairs of your head are all numbered.'

__ Luke 12:7a NKJV

When I used to draw comic strips (I know I'll get back to it one day), before starting any new comic strip I would take blank pages and draw each character. I would put details into their hair, the color of their hair, their eyes, the shape of their body, their facial expressions when sad, angry, crying, laughing etc. I would also spend hours in my mind imaging everything about them. One day it just dawned on me that if I spend so much effort for characters who remain on paper, how much more God for us in whom He breathed life.

God put love and detail in every part of you, including your hair. The color, texture, porosity and type of your hair aren't coincidences. He chose it intentionally and He designed you like that and considered it to be very good.

Instead of seeing your hair as something difficult to manage, see it as God's gift to you and ask Him to give you tips and insights on how to care for it and even on how to style it. As for me for example, there are so many ingredients on earth but He's The One who inspires me on ingredients to use for hair masks and hair oils specifically for me. Additionally, before I style my hair, I ask Him which hairstyle to go for.

When you stop seeing your hair as a burden and you start seeing it as a gift from God, instead of trying to hide it or destroy it for it to look like other people's hair, you'll begin to love it and inquire of The Lord on ways to take care of it. Your hair will then grow longer, stronger and healthier all to the glory of God's Name.

Prayer to love your hair

Father Lord God Almighty, my Creator, I thank You for being intentional in choosing my hair type, porosity and texture. Please forgive me for when I didn't love my hair and for when I almost destroyed it by trying to look like others. Please Lord, teach me to love my hair the way it is and teach me to care for it the way You originally intended for me to care for it, in Jesus Christ's Name. Amen

Perhaps you just said this prayer and you felt the desire to have a deep intimate relationship with God you can also say the following prayer:

Prayer to have a deep intimate relationship with God [9]

Lord Jesus, I know that I am a sinner, I have sinned against You and I ask for Your forgiveness. I believe You love me so much that You died for my sins and rose from the dead. I make the decision today to turn from my sins and I invite You to come into my life, change my nature from a nature of sin to a nature of righteousness, set me free, give me a new nature, transform my life so that I live a holy life. I choose from this day forward to love You, to obey You, to humble myself under the mighty hand of God, to practice self-denial, to put You first and to live above the world. I want to live a holy life which glorifies God's Name. I surrender myself completely to You Lord, spirit, soul and body. I choose today to trust and follow You as my Lord and Saviour. My life is Yours. I choose to obey You. Amen

CONTACT INFORMATION

For any inquiries, coaching and partnership opportunities, feel free to contact the author at zoeschooloflife@gmail.com

Most of the products mentioned above can be found on my amazon store front https://www.amazon.com/shop/victoriaeyog

REFERENCES

1. Chang CJ, O'Brien KM, Keil AP, Gaston SA, Jackson CL, Sandler DP, et al. Use of Straighteners and Other Hair Products and Incident Uterine Cancer. J Natl Cancer Inst. 2022 Dec 8;114(12):1636–45.

2. Eberle CE, Sandler DP, Taylor KW, White AJ. Hair dye and chemical straightener use and breast cancer risk in a large US population of black and white women. Int J Cancer. 2020 Jul 15;147(2):383–91.

3. Stiel L, Adkins-Jackson PB, Clark P, Mitchell E, Montgomery S. A review of hair product use on breast cancer risk in African American women. Cancer Med. 2016 Mar;5(3):597–604.

4. White AJ, Gregoire AM, Taylor KW, Eberle C, Gaston S, O'Brien KM, et al. Adolescent use of hair dyes, straighteners and perms in relation to breast cancer risk. Int J Cancer. 2021 May 1;148(9):2255–63.

5. Bertrand KA, Delp L, Coogan PF, Cozier YC, Lenzy YM, Rosenberg L, et al. Hair relaxer use and risk of uterine cancer in the Black Women's Health Study. Environmental Research. 2023 Dec 15;239:117228.

6. Hatsbach de Paula JN, Basílio FMA, Mulinari-Brenner FA. Effects of chemical straighteners on the hair shaft and scalp. An Bras Dermatol. 2022;97(2):193–203.

7. How To Determine Your Hair Porosity [Internet]. Cliphair UK. 2023 [cited 2024 Mar 1]. Available from: https://www.cliphair.co.uk/blogs/hair-blog/how-to-determine-your-hair-porosity

8. The Maximum Hydration Method: 6 Steps to Soft Natural Hair [Internet]. Byrdie. [cited 2024 Feb 24]. Available from: https://www.byrdie.com/maximum-hydration-method-4767940

9. victoriaeyog. Salvation 101: The Necessity of an entire renovation of character and life for all who would enter Heaven [Internet]. Mission For Jesus. 2021 [cited 2024 Feb 24]. Available from: https://missionforjesus.blog/salvation-101-the-necessity-of-an-entire-renovation-of-character-and-life-for-all-who-would-enter-heaven

ABOUT THE AUTHOR

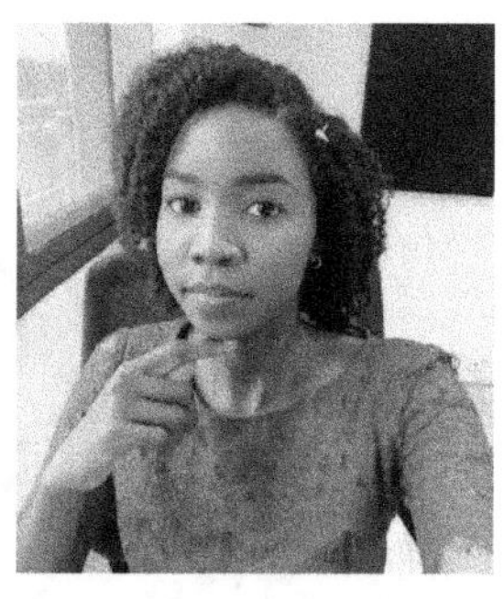 Victoria Eyog Tang Nlend is a Christian woman, a wife, a mother, a Doctor of Pharmacy. She's the founder of Zoe the School of Life. She is a natural hair advocate and a hair & skin beauty coach for black and African-American women. She was born in Cameroon, and she is passionate about making women in Cameroon and worldwide love and embrace their God-given natural hair as a crown of glory. She teaches black women how to grow and maintain healthy, shiny, lustrous and voluminous natural hair with simplistic yet efficacious well-kept secrets and natural products derived from the Cameroonian and African culture. Her tips have helped black women to transition from relaxed to natural hair smoothly and to (re)grow healthy and long natural hair after damage caused by harsh chemicals, relaxers, heat and poor styling habits.